# Mindfulness for the 5:2 Diet

Lose weight faster, feel happier, take control by eating mindfully

## Polly Fielding

ISBN-13: 978-1500732615
ISBN-10:1500732613

**Author's Note**:

Whilst every effort has been taken to ensure the accuracy of everything in this book, the author apologises in the event of any mistakes being found

# Other books by Polly Fielding

The 5:2 Diet Made eZy

The 5:2 Vegetarian Diet Made eZy

Single Serving Recipes To Soothe Arthritis

Single Serving Vegetarian Recipes To Soothe Arthritis

Delicious Vegetarian Diabetic Meals For One

Vegetarian Recipes For One To Lower Blood Pressure

And This Is My Adopted Daughter

A Mind To Be Free

Crossing The Borderline

Letting Go

Breaking The Silence

Missing Factor (A personal experience of haemophilia)

Going In Seine

Nurturing Compassion

Moments Of Mindfulness

Time For Mindfulness

A Veritable Smorgasbord

**www.pollyfielding.com**

This book is dedicated to Seán whose mindful, compassionate and insightful approach greatly enriched my life

# Contents

# Introduction

Just as there is a great deal of interest in the 5:2 diet (or fast diet, as it is also called) and why it works so well for so many people, there is a steadily growing curiosity and discussion about mindfulness in the media. This is hardly surprising when you begin to understand what an exciting and exceedingly simple concept it is and how using it can make a huge difference to your daily life.

And anyone of any age can do it with minimal effort!

So by combining the healthy 5:2 way of eating with mindfulness you have an excellent recipe for success. My aim in this book is to explain exactly how to make them work for you in easy, practical, straightforward steps.

# A brief explanation of the 5:2 Diet

 Although some of you may well be familiar with the principles of the 5:2 method of eating, for those who have just come across it, I will summarise what it is and why it works.

Each week, for any two days of your choice, you reduce your calorie intake to a quarter of the recommended daily allowance - which means 500 calories for women and 600 for men (it might not sound like much but it's amazing what you can actually consume for that amount).   On the other five days you eat normally.

Where this diet scores over others is that it is extremely manageable in both the long as well as short term because, apart from the fact that no food is forbidden, you only have to stick to it on two days.  Before too long, your knowledge of the calorie content of different foods will become second nature to you just as riding a bike or learning to drive (can you remember how that seemed quite a lot to remember at the start?).

There is plenty of scientific research, both with animals and increasingly with humans, to provide us with sufficient justification for believing that by restricting our calorie consumption twice weekly we can achieve more than weight loss and protect ourselves against developing obesity-linked conditions such as diabetes type II, heart disease, and some cancers. We can also help to protect ourselves against age-related brain diseases, like Alzheimer's, which affect such a large number of people.

With a few exceptions, we all have the IGF-1 hormone (an insulin-related growth hormone) inside our bodies, which helped us to reach adult height but, unfortunately, has a tendency to increase in amount as we age and can become detrimental to health. 5:2 eating results in a lowering of the level and its drop triggers DNA repair genes to begin undoing some of the damage that has already been done to existing cells.

In addition to the distinct possibility of a longer, healthier existence, plenty of evidence is emerging to bear out a variety of further benefits to this productive lifestyle - increased energy, lowered appetite on the five normal eating days, improvement of mood, improved body image, higher self esteem, better food choices among them.

And taking sensible amounts of regular exercise inevitably speeds up the gains mentioned.

The 5:2 is a widely recommended style of eating; in fact there are many doctors who have adopted it. However, no medical professional would advocate this regime for children, people with a serious eating disorder, anyone who is pregnant or breast-feeding, has diabetes or indeed any serious illness. If you are at all doubtful about whether you have a condition which would make this diet unsuitable for you, please seek your GP's advice before beginning it.

# Celia's story

When I met up with a school friend whom I hadn't seen for years, it soon became clear that, although she tried to appear happy, she was deeply troubled. After we'd chatted for a while she poured out her unhappiness. She began by telling me that she'd recently been to her GP, who'd given her an ultimatum. Over the next couple of hours she gave me the complete picture.

Until she was eight Celia (not her real name) had been a slim, active, happy outgoing child. Then her parents got divorced. She and her younger brother lived with their mother and rarely saw their father from that time onwards.

She can remember feeling that somehow it must have been her fault that they had split up. It was only years afterwards that she discovered that her dad had been having an affair which had led to the breakdown of the marriage.

Her mum and grandmother were very good cooks. She said that she'd always enjoyed their appetizing meals and homemade bread and cakes so it wasn't difficult to follow their rule of eating everything on her plate. Except that now she began to have second helpings, particularly of desserts. She also started spending all her pocket money on sweets and was often rewarded with candies for good behaviour at home.

As she dropped all after-school sport activities, preferring to absorb herself in books, her weight increased until she became an easy target for the class bully who began to make fun of her size. So she took refuge in food, finding that eating made her feel better at least temporarily.

As a teenager she ate a lot of fast food whenever she went out with her friends. But, whilst they didn't seem to get fatter on it, Celia ballooned still further. She noticed that the boys seemed to go out with them whilst she got over-looked, despite her constant efforts to look attractive, so she determined to diet and lose the excessive extra pounds she'd put on over the years.

She tried one diet after another, but each one felt too punishing, depriving her of most of her favourite foods for too long, so after dropping several pounds she'd give up trying. Then a couple of months would pass before she'd once again enthusiastically begin the yoyo-dieting cycle.

In her late twenties she met and married someone who was more interested in Celia as a person than her steadily mounting weight gain though, in order to fit into the wedding dress she'd set her heart on, she went on yet another quick-fix solution to achieve her goal.

After the birth of each of her three children she added on yet more pounds. Then, as her husband's business took him to various parts of the globe for increasingly longer stretches at a time, she sought even greater refuge in food to console herself in his absence.

When their youngest child flew the nest to begin a flat-share whilst he was at university, although Celia was happy for him she missed him dreadfully even pining for his loud music, messy room and strange collection of friends!

Her waist expanded until she could no longer fit comfortably into her size 20 clothes; her self esteem and poor body image plummeted to rock bottom as the scales shot up to two hundred and twenty-five pounds. She felt terribly unhappy and ashamed of herself. It had now got to the point, she confided, where she avoided looking in a mirror to do her hair.

The final straw for Celia was when she waddled off to the doctor to find out why she was constantly tired, had difficulty with her breathing whenever she walked any distance and never seemed to have an ounce of energy. Her GP had laid it straight on the line, telling her in no uncertain terms that she was definitely obese and that, unless she drastically changed her eating patterns and began exercising, she was quite literally eating herself into a very early grave.

The dietician her doctor referred her to had helped her examine carefully the kind of things she was eating and introduced her to good, healthy food options. But she found that she was still overeating and feeling the need to consume large amounts of food.  She said she knew she must do something about it, but was getting desperate because her desire for food was so all-consuming and felt overwhelming at times, particularly for anything sweet...

After listening to her dilemma  about how vital it was to her health that she lost the weight accumulated over the years and kept it off,  I began telling her about the serious wake-up call I'd  needed to spur me into looking closely at not only what I ate on a daily basis but why.

 Then I described the style of eating that I'd been following for nearly two years, called the 5:2 diet.

She was truly sceptical when I said that she could still eat her favourite foods, but seemed encouraged by the fact that I'd already been following it for such a long time and had not only managed to lose unwanted pounds but also found it easy to stick to.  She fully intended to carry on with it indefinitely.

 I told her that the diet was only a part of my strong resolve to make radical changes to how, what and when I ate. Because, even though once I'd checked with my GP that it was ok for me to start the 5:2 and realised that this way of eating actually did work and was far more practical and realistic than any other diet I'd ever attempted, I still felt discontented, restless and  generally dissatisfied with my life.

 So in my search to help myself to feel happier, I'd begun a

course in mindfulness.

I told her about the light bulb that came on in my head during my study of this concept and the clear realisation kicking in that, for most of my life, food had been my closest friend and ally, that I had been using food in an effort to satisfy and push down painful emotions. When I'd reflected on what and when I'd eaten and the times I had indulged most, it became obvious to me that I'd spent years habitually resorting to food in an attempt to compensate for the way I felt.

It had become instinctive to eat whenever I was upset, bored, lonely, angry, resentful, stressed, fearful... And it almost always seemed to help - briefly. For a short period of time my mood would improve, only to crash as time passed and I'd added guilt, shame and self-blame to my store of negativity. After all, I could not hold anyone else responsible for what I chose to put into my mouth.

Yet it wasn't for lack of trying to be a slimmer, healthier, more positive person that I had ended up fat, tired and unhappy. I was desperately doing everything I thought would help me. Then when 'my best' wasn't good enough I was using it as a stick to beat myself which, of course, made me feel worse still.

I'd never faced up to my feelings in a constructive, helpful, positive manner but had used food as a comfort or reward instead; I'd covered up and tried to make myself happier in the only manner I knew how. But in so doing, I'd never really stopped for long enough to learn how to get to a comfortable place inside me and find a different, infinitely more satisfying solution.

But I said that it hadn't been an overnight process; no ingrained habit is that easy to break. It had taken me a fair amount of time and practice but, just like the discovery of a new approach to eating, I'd become sufficiently interested to put a reasonable degree of thought and effort into it.

I explained about how once mindfulness had become an integral part of each day, it was the most natural thing in the world to apply it to the preparation of food and eating it. When I became aware that I was an emotional eater I was able to make the much-needed changes and take control of why, when, what, and how I ate and break the vicious cycle that had been so damaging to my health. Food had now become a source of delight and thorough enjoyment.

Celia began to look somewhat more hopeful as I talked about how I used mindfulness to help me overcome any difficulties with my 5:2 eating pattern; told her about the benefits and the simplicity behind them and how they had dramatically changed my life for the better, both physically and mentally.

I told her that I also used to feel helpless and out of control, assured her that if I could change my relationship with food I was confident  she could too,   As our evening together drew to a close and we exchanged phone numbers, I suggested we keep in touch and pledged my support.

I will tell you more about Celia later.

# Mindfulness in a nutshell

There is nothing mysterious about mindfulness.  In fact, it is a simple concept which, just like the restriction of food intake, is not recent.  Both ideas have been practised for many years.

Mindfulness can actually be summed up in one sentence, though I will describe it at greater length so that it becomes more readily understood.

**Being mindful means to be fully aware of each moment, accepting it just as it is right now, with compassion and without judgement.**

I'll take each component in turn.

Living in the present entails moment-to-moment noticing of what is happening inside and around you.  Although this may sound like I'm stating the downright obvious, most of us have a tendency to multi-task; our attention is frequently not entirely focussed on doing one thing at a time.

So whilst I'm typing I might also be drinking a cup of coffee, worrying about my son, gazing at passers-by out of the window and listening to the news on the radio.  Is it any wonder that, whilst I continue trying to do five things simultaneously, I keep losing my train of thought?  And, frequently we aren't even really conscious that we're engaged in attempting to do several completely unconnected things at once. Such unawareness can lead to feeling incredibly stressed, pressurised, exhausted and irritable.

The ever-changing highly technological age we live in nowadays has numerous advantages to daily life but a downside is that, with the many different options available like smart phones, social networking, emails... we can be too easily distracted.

When you become aware, though, of lots of things happening in you – the way you feel, the constant self-chatter in your head - going on at the same time as things that are going on around you, it creates a spaciousness. This mindful space gives you more options like choosing a particular activity to concentrate your entire attention on right here, right now, or just deciding to watch and *be* rather than *do* anything at all.

You cease to miss out on the finer details of a task and become far more effective in tackling something. It's rather like waking up after a long sleep, seeing everything in a fresh light as though for the very first time.

When I began to practise mindfulness I saw colours more brightly, patterns in my rugs that I could not have described if asked to do so unless they'd been in front of me, plants in my garden that I didn't even know were there, had a heightened curiosity, an interest in everything and developed a stronger appreciation of people, of life itself, opened up to new possibilities...

The present is where you are, there's nowhere else to be, nowhere to go. You are already there!

Acceptance of how things actually are in this moment is another important aspect of mindfulness.

 If you push negative thoughts away, trying to avoid what you are experiencing if it feels unpleasant, they have a habit of returning time after time - the very act of resisting makes their persistence extremely probable. Similarly, loads of energy can be used up and wasted by seeking to hold onto anything that occurs which gives you a pleasant sensation.

 The phrase that springs to mind 'It is as it is', so not necessarily how you would wish the situation to be, not always fair. But as soon as you acknowledge and allow things to be exactly as they are for the moment, when you stop fighting to change them you can begin to shift your perception of them or, if it's possible, take considered action over what needs to be done.

 Basically, it is by recognition and acceptance that you can make positive changes inside or outside yourself, or in the case of something you are not able to change – decrease feelings of helplessness and lack of control by taking the decision to accept its reality instead of futilely working incessantly to make it otherwise.

A further essential element of mindfulness is compassion, in particular compassion for yourself. I think that, generally, people find it much easier to be kind to others than to themselves. When I find myself being really critical of myself, thinking unkind thoughts about something I've felt, done or said – and it took me ages to realise how much harsh, critical self-talk actually went on in my mind! – I ask myself what I could say to a friend who was thinking such thoughts, in order to figure out nicer ways to speak to myself in my head. I find that, in an instant, both the tone and words I use change for the better.

When you start to listen to your own internal monologue you will begin to see how the manner in which you talk to yourself, countless times a day, powerfully affects how you see yourself and the world. And, once you become kinder to yourself, it follows naturally that you will view others with increased compassion. You will become more sensitive to their needs as well as your own which will inevitably influence your response to them.

Finally, but no less importantly, is the non-judgemental part of mindfulness, which is not the same as failure to acknowledge anything as harmful or helpful, nor is it a lack of discernment.

Clearly, everyone has to make a variety of decisions for themselves and other people in the course of their everyday life, based on their knowledge and experience.

When you are being mindful it is about seeing the facts and separating them from your opinion of them. It's standing back sufficiently to observe and patiently watch the automatic judgements you make about yourself and others so that you can get an altogether clearer perspective. You will find, if you put this into practice, that you will be considerably less inclined to end up mentally beating yourself up, or them.

## A straightforward guide to mindful eating and drinking

We all need to eat – it is a natural instinctive activity to satisfy hunger that we are born with and, like many other instincts, it is pleasurable.

What is not inherent from birth is a craving for food when we aren't hungry. You only have to watch babies to realise that when they need feeding they cry but as soon as their hunger is satisfied they stop eating.   When you have fed a baby it will turn away if you offer more, knowing that it's had enough.

Somewhere along the line as we grow up we often lose this balance.  We develop unconscious habits which can alter our relationship with food quite dramatically.  And this unawareness is resulting in growing levels of obesity, disease and unhappiness in the western world.

It doesn't have to be like this though.  We are all capable of change; whilst we continue to draw breath it's never too late.   And you have already taken an important step to transform your way of eating by choosing the 5:2 diet. You were aware of previously eating unhealthily, you knew that that your weight gain was a problem and that you had to do something constructive about it.

Although you think far more consciously about food on your two diet days and make better decisions about when and what to eat, you may still find that you are feeling hungry at times.

But are you always really hungry for food or is there another reason for this feeling? Looking closely and working out what is truly triggering this apparent need to head for the fridge or nearest cupboard can give you greater choice over how you respond to this discomfort inside you.

When you get what distinctly feels like a cue to eat, pause for long enough to ask yourself if this is your body telling you that it requires food or whether perhaps your mind is misinterpreting the signal you are getting.

It could be that you need a drink because you are thirsty – at times hunger can be mistaken for thirst. Try having a glass of cold water which has the plus of being completely free of calories. Add a few mint or basil leaves or a couple of drops of lemon juice, if that makes it more palatable for you. But make your action of drinking this essential life-giving fluid different this time from how you might usually do it, by experiencing it mindfully with the following exercise:-

- Sit down, being aware as you do so where your body is making contact with the chair and how that feels.
- Take a sip of water. Let it remain in your mouth for a few moments. Notice its coolness, any flavour and changes in temperature as you continue to hold it.

- As you swallow, feel the sensation of the fluid passing down your throat, the sound as it disappears, how your mouth feels afterwards.
- Do this with each sip, watching as your thoughts stray somewhere else but not getting caught up in them and not criticizing yourself for having them, then returning your attention to the process as before.

By drinking slowly as if it's something you've never done, in the manner I've just described, you are using moment-to-moment mindfulness. It's that easy! And obviously, you can decide to do this exercise with any type of drink you choose for your diet days (hydration with plenty of liquid is vital for every cell in the body). You can have a new experience every time you practise it. I particularly like the taste of lemon green tea which has just one calorie.

If, when you have finished the water, you still feel that you want to eat, possibly craving something sweet, ask yourself if what you are feeling is in fact an emotional reaction.

Are you bored, tired, sad, lonely, stressed out, fearful, depressed, anxious, angry...?

Food and drink cannot truly satisfy these emotions, they need to be responded to differently, firstly by accepting that they are there and then by finding a way to deal with their causes. If they are not recognised and handled appropriately, if you are denying them by using food to avoid them, to cover them up or feed them, you will make yourself feel even worse by adding guilt and shame to the store of negativity.

When you are physically hungry, it is less likely to be a sudden impulse to eat and more of a rumbling and aching in your stomach, which begins to hurt if you don't eat. Eventually, if you continue to ignore the symptoms, your concentration wanes, you may get shaky and light-headed and become unbearably irritable. And if you wait for too long, you will be tempted to eat more than your body needs. So it's important to listen to your body and be sensitive to its requirements.

Additionally, knowing when you've had enough food is necessary. But, it takes time for the stomach to tell your head that it's had a sufficient amount of food on account of the fact that the digestive hormones your gastrointestinal tract secretes take a while to get transmitted to the brain. So the speed at which you consume your meal will determine whether or not you can be effective in deciding when to stop eating. If you eat reasonably slowly you can find that you feel full more quickly, even though you are eating less.

When you eat mindfully, you will be in tune with your body and meet its needs healthily and with true enjoyment.

I used to be so distracted when I ate. I'd grab breakfast on the run, rush through what I was eating whilst thinking about all the things I had to do later or stressing over something I'd forgotten to do. To be honest, I hardly ever paid attention to what I devoured. With so many pressures from within and around me – deadlines to meet, targets to achieve, constant demands to do something, be somewhere... I'd cook meals in 'automatic mode' or snack thoughtlessly whilst watching television or browsing on my laptop, scarcely noting either the process of preparation or properly tasting whatever I put in my mouth. Time seemed in such short supply that eating was just another facet of the relentlessly fast pace of my daily, stressful treadmill.

It was only when I stopped to consider why I felt constantly exhausted, too worn out to do much at the end of each evening apart from fall into bed to snatch a few hours sleep before stepping onto another uncomfortable roller-coaster ride of a day, that it struck me that I was trying to do too many things at a time. In my frantic efforts to achieve, to get a lot done and feel I hadn't wasted a moment, life was passing me by and I had no idea of what I was missing. Listening to the phrase at the beginning of Paul Simon's 59th Street Bridge Song: 'Slow down, you move too fast', I reflected – that's me!

The first thing I had to do when I began reprogramming my brain patterns was to stop, breathe with awareness and then slow down.

On your next diet day it's worth trying this next exercise

for a minute or two, shortly before you prepare your first meal. You can do it sitting, standing or lying down:-

- If you are sitting have both feet on the floor. Close your eyes if that feels comfortable.
- Place the palm of one hand on your chest and your other hand over your belly (just under your ribs) then inhale through your nose, slowly and deeply, noticing as you do so which of your hands is the first to move - if the hand on your chest moves first you are breathing shallowly, something many people do.
- Keeping your hands where they are take another slow breath in, making sure that it begins in your belly (feeling it slowly expand like a balloon filling with air) before moving up to your chest.
- Holding your breath, count steadily to 5 (one and two and three...).
- Breathe out slowly, through parted lips, until all the air has been emptied from your lungs.
- Wait for the count of 5.
- Repeat the above for several further breaths.

This simple technique, besides giving your blood a healthy boost of oxygen, will help you to feel relaxed and be in a calmer frame of mind to focus on preparing something to eat.

As I am writing this specifically to use with your two calorie-restricted days, I am going to make the assumption that you will already have shopped with your diet days in mind. It's worth pointing out here that it's important to glance at labels on packaging, noting what comes high up on the list of contents. By law, besides stating the product's calorie content, manufacturers are obliged to show the ingredients in decreasing order of amounts, the ones nearest the top being more plentiful than the rest. There is, therefore, the power for you to make more informed choices about what to buy.

However you have decided to structure your diet days - whether to space your calories over the day, spread them across two meals or just have one, is up to you. My personal preference is to have a reasonable sized breakfast, a light snack for lunch and a fairly substantial supper early in the evening. I have found this to be the method that suits me best but how you choose to do it is entirely up to you. As with the practice of mindful eating, there is no right or wrong way; when you engage with food with greater attention you will find a route that is best for you.

I have selected a recipe from the final section of this book to use to illustrate an application of mindful awareness to preparing and eating a meal when you know you will not be too pressed for time - there's little point, for instance, in attempting this when in half an hour you have to pick the children up from school! You need to allow yourself enough space to do it; otherwise you'll be unlikely to try the same sort of thing ever again.

Please read the instructions that follow the recipe before beginning the preparation, to first give yourself the overall picture.

## Roasted Tomatoes, Red onions and Mushrooms

## 71 Calories

## Ingredients

1 small plum tomato, chopped into small chunks

½ small sweet or red onion, sliced thinly

42g (1½ oz) mushrooms, sliced thickly

1 tsp. olive oil

2 tsp. red wine vinegar

1 tsp. fresh basil, finely chopped

Ground black pepper

## Method

- Preheat oven to $200^0$C/$400^0$F/Gas mark 6

- In a large bowl, mix tomato chunks with onion & mushroom slices
- Add oil, vinegar, basil & mix thoroughly with vegetables
- Season with black pepper to taste
- Line a baking tray with non-stick foil
- Spread vegetable mixture onto tray
- Roast vegetables until onion slices are browned & rest of vegetables are tender, keeping track when they are cooking to ensure that vegetables do not shrivel up. (approx.15 - 20 minutes)
- Serve hot

## Mindful preparation

- Once you've switched on the oven to heat up, choose your cutlery and plate with attention (your portion of food will look better on a smaller surface).
- Take time over setting your place at a table. A small vase of flowers can make it more pleasing to the eye.
- When you select your raw ingredients for this meal appreciate the colours, think about their source - the farmer that planted the seeds, the rain and sun that nourished their growth, how they got to your

grocery store, why you selected them.

- As you slice and chop the vegetables reflect on the movement of your hand, how the vegetables feel to the touch, what they look like as you cut them. If other thoughts pop into your head acknowledge them and gently return your focus to what you are doing.
- Notice their colour and softness or crunchiness as you are slicing and chopping.
- Watch the changes in juiciness as you cut into the tomato.
- Pay attention to the smell released by slicing into the onion.
- Listen to the sound your knife makes on the chopping board.
- Look closely at the variety of patterns inside the vegetables.

## Eating with mindfulness

- Make sure, before you sit down to enjoy what you've cooked, that the TV, radio, phone and other distractions are turned off, that all you need to concentrate on right now is eating; this exercise works best, when you first try it, on your own and in silence - something that's in short supply, this side of the grave!
- Look at the meal on your plate before you

commence eating; your combination of colours, the various shapes, the aromas wafting towards you, noting the increase of saliva this produces (though don't wait so long that your food gets cold and less appetising!).

- Notice what you select to eat first, which muscles you use to raise it to your mouth and pause, before starting to bite it, just long enough to notice how it feels there.
- As you chew it, do so slowly with a curious awareness of the taste, flavour, texture, temperature, any changes in them and where in your mouth they register most strongly.
- When you swallow, feel the sensation, hear the sound it makes. Is there an aftertaste in your mouth?
- Repeat this process with each further morsel of food.
- Observe when your thoughts wander off, not judging them to be good or bad, merely thoughts passing through your mind like clouds - but be kind to yourself if you do get hooked on them for a while – refocusing on the present when you realise this is happening.
- Be attentive, before you leave the table, to how your body is feeling and any emotions you may be experiencing.
- Then reflect on how you have nourished and taken care of yourself.

# Why it works so well

The exercises in the previous section are examples of the vast variety of possibilities available for nourishing your mind as well as your body on your diet days – ways to introduce you to eating with mindfulness. Your own creative nature will guide you, in time, towards alternative approaches to tackling your personal eating patterns.

What's important is to utilise your five senses to the full; savouring food with touch, taste, smell, hearing and sight to enhance your experience of it.

There is nothing complicated about a meal prepared like this and eaten with sensitive, sensory attention. It is simply the purposeful and conscious awareness that you are bringing to it which is perhaps different from how you might have often habitually eaten.

And you will find that, though of course you don't eat everything in the day this slowly and with such a measured degree of attention, it will, nevertheless, soon become a habit to appreciate and enjoy more fully whatever you put into your mouth. Mealtimes turn into sources of delight and sheer pleasure.

But most probably, you'll become more adventurous, as I did, in experimenting with combinations of food that you had never thought of; perhaps discover foods from cultures that you've not tried previously. What you eat can sometimes be totally new and exciting.

There are other advantages to the practice of mindful eating which will encourage you to want to do it more frequently, though possibly not as slowly as the first time.

For starters, the net result of the slower-paced timing of your consumption ensures that you'll be better able to know when you've eaten enough. You will learn to recognize intuitively when you are satiated because you are in harmony with your body and listening to what it is trying to tell you; regaining, quite naturally, the art of being in tune with your physical needs that you had when you were born.

And when you've applied this method a few times you will start to modify how, when and what you eat on non calorie-restricted days. Feeling in greater control you'll be considerably less likely to binge.

It's worth noting here that, to increase your chances of success, it makes sense, on diet and non-diet days, to keep healthy foodstuff towards the front of the shelves in your fridge and cupboards so that's what you see the moment you open the door.

A bowl of varying colours of fruit looks good and is a healthy option both if you fancy a snack on your five days of normal eating and to choose for a shorter mindful eating practice. Moreover, a greater variety of colours indicates a broader nutritional intake.

Your digestion is sure to respond better when you eat more healthily and ingest plenty of fruit and vegetables which, in addition to tasting nice, meet your body's need for fibre, antioxidants and other essential nutrients.

However, that is not the entire story, because whatever you eat, you could still find yourself suffering from uncomfortable digestive problems like bloating, unless the food has been thoroughly broken up before it passes into the digestive tract. Chewing well enables food to break down completely and combine effectively with digestive enzymes before we even get as far as swallowing it.

A further reason why eating with mindful intention works so well is that you'll gradually develop a lasting, balanced, healthy, satisfying attitude towards yourself as well as to your food.

If you decide to choose a calorie-laden or fatty item, knowing that it's fine to have this occasional treat you won't spoil it by overlaying it with negative emotions such as shame and guilt.

As you steadily and healthily lose weight and relish the act of eating you begin to feel better about yourself, your sense of self-worth increases along with confidence and higher energy levels and you reach the realisation that it's worthwhile continuing on this path.

And now to return to Celia. We kept in contact intermittently with brief phone calls over the next six months before meeting up again. I was amazed and delighted at the transformation.  She approached me smiling, considerably slimmer and positively glowing with health and enthusiasm.

 She then told me how different she felt from the last time we met and why.

 She'd begun shopping for the 5:2 diet the following day when her doctor assured her it was fine to go ahead provided she was sensible about it.  Then she had psyched herself up to get started at the end of that week.

 She said that at first it had felt terribly strange and she'd initially suffered a lot from her usual food cravings, headaches and other symptoms.  But she remembered that I'd told her it wouldn't necessarily be plain sailing and that it was worthwhile persevering as there were ways of overcoming these obstacles without being harsh on herself.

She did feel extremely hungry in the beginning, as her body tried to adapt to a much lower intake than usual, but the thought that the next day she would not be restricting her calories to this extent consoled her somewhat and kept her going for the time being.

And knowing that water before her meal would help her feel less hungry, she got used to moving to the tap instead of the fridge and having a drink more regularly throughout the day without waiting until she felt thirsty.  In fact, when her head began to ache, instead of rushing straight to the medicine cabinet for painkillers, she'd found that a glass of water often solved the problem.

However, on a non-diet day her resolve would weaken further and she'd quickly revert to overeating.

It was mainly the fear that giving up could mean that she might not live to see her teenage children become fully-fledged adults that spurred her on. Whenever she was severely tempted to eat a huge tub of ice cream, a big bar of chocolate, half a packet of biscuits or similar things she was so used to eating regularly, she'd pause to examine why she wanted them. Gradually, she came to the conclusion that she'd been comfort eating on a regular basis for so many years that, understandably, this wasn't going to be an easy ride. The more she considered what her apparent hunger was about, the greater her realisation that much of the time she was trying to appease and avoid her true emotions by stuffing them down and trying to stifle them with food.

She'd eaten alone sometimes on a diet day so that she didn't have to converse with anyone and be distracted by what they or she were saying. And it was during these times of eating with mindful attention that she found herself less caught up in thinking about the past or the future and considerably more connected with the present. She told me that it had been then that she began to enjoy food rather than continually use it as a substitute for identifying and coping with her emotions.

She recognised that one of her long-held habits was to take total responsibility when things went wrong in relationships, particularly with her husband. She'd always ended up blaming herself completely rather than appreciating that she merely needed to hold herself to account for her own part and not for what others said or did.

And remembering the importance of kindness she'd then begun to make allowances for her own as well as other people's lapses knowing that none of us is supposed to be perfect. She had learnt to apply some compassion to herself.

She said she was unbelievably shocked when she'd listened carefully to her self-talk. She would never have spoken to anyone else using the hard, mocking, critical tone and unforgiving words she heard repeated over and over again in her mind such as' You're *still* too fat!' and 'How could you be so stupid?'.

If she felt lonely she'd pop in on an elderly neighbour who lived on her own and was glad of a chat. When she was bored she decided to go for walk or do some gardening.

Now when she chose to have ice cream, she did so deliberately and was contented with a small amount with none of the guilt and unhappiness that had previously accompanied it.

She'd learnt how to connect with herself healthily and

mindfully, which had led to a change in how she related to food.  Her 5:2 lifestyle had become easier; much more manageable and effective with the result that she was continuing steadily to lose weight (she'd already shed thirty-nine pounds, she announced proudly), and her breathing difficulties had totally disappeared .  She felt energised enough to go swimming a couple of times each week and had joined a yoga class; best of all she felt happier in her own skin.

She told me that shopping for clothes was something she'd come to enjoy; feeling better about herself, her perception of how she looked had improved and she felt incentivised to buy colourful clothing to show off her new figure instead of the drab, shapeless items that she used to hide behind.

And a recent medical check up had shown that the diet, together with her new approach to herself and her life, had paid off.  On top of the obvious weight loss, her blood pressure and blood test results were now normal and she was no longer at imminent risk of diabetes.

## Positive spin-offs from using this approach

Eating the 5:2 way gives you the freedom over when and what you choose to consume. And factoring in mindfulness helps you to watch how you feel inside and understand your motivation to eat, in addition to gaining an increased appreciation of food.

However, there are a variety of other benefits which are offshoots from your lower calorie days and the time, care and attention you are allowing yourself.

The efforts you make for awareness will creep into other times when food is involved. So, during the remainder of the week, you'll inevitably find yourself making choices that are healthier for you and eating less haphazardly.

You will pretty soon find your attitude in all areas of your life changing too.

For instance, take a conversation you are having with someone. If the other person is speaking we're often not listening quite as helpfully as we might be; we can hear what they are saying to us yet, simultaneously, be thinking of what we are going to reply when they stop or judging the content of their words, perhaps deciding that they are right or wrong in their opinions. And have you ever kept flipping back and forth, thinking or worrying about something else completely, as you remain broadly in contact with the gist of whatever they are expressing?  I know I have!

With your developing perceptiveness you will sometimes recognise that this is happening as you converse.  This flags up the need to let go of trying to work out what answer you are going to give before you reach that point and allows you the space to listen, without hijacking your ability to do so, with openness and tolerance.

Everyday, ordinary routine activities - showering when you can really feel and smell  the soap or gel, be soothed by the sensation of warm water on your skin...cleaning your teeth, walking, breathing, anything you do -  become opportunities for the simplicity of mindful practice.

 And, like anything else you do frequently, being with the present moment gets to be a habit; one which can significantly lower your stress levels, enable you to savour pleasurable experiences more fully and relieve the relentless pressure you may otherwise put on yourself to strive too hard.

You'll find you have more of an open curiosity about life and what it has to offer, cope more effectively with adversity and have a greater connection with other people.

Being more self-compassionate you will feel better in and about yourself, achieve more...

I could continue, but I know you'll be able to add your own

examples because when you slow down and go with the flow they will arise naturally.

# Easy recipes for your diet days

# Notes

❖ Although these recipes are single-serving, you can, of course, double the quantities for two.

❖ I have tried to include a variety to suit different tastes and cater for vegetarian as well as non-vegetarian.

❖ With regards to cooking spray, my preference is for 1-cal olive oil but there is a variety of low calorie sprays on the market for you to choose from.

❖ Stevia is a useful product since, unlike many sugar substitutes, it is entirely natural – derived from the leaves of the South American plant of that name. It is very sweet; if you would normally use a teaspoon of sugar, a third of that amount will give you an equal degree of sweetness. Stevia is marketed under a variety of brand names and is widely available.

❖ I felt that to mention washing fruit and vegetables, except where specifically stated, was unnecessary since I am sure that you do that anyway.

❖ It could be worth investing in a set of smallish attractive plates to add to the presentation and appearance of your reduced portion sizes; this can have a pleasing psychological as well as visual impact.

❖ Using smaller cutlery can also help to slow down your consumption of a meal, for example with a teaspoon you will put less at a time into your mouth.

❖ If you want to slow your eating pace even further, you could occasionally try eating any solid food with chopsticks.

❖ I have listed recipes under breakfast, lunch and supper headings but, of course, you can mix and match – they don't have to be defined by the titles.

❖ Whichever recipes you choose and whenever you decide to use them, I wish you a pleasurable experience.

# BREAKFASTS

# Creamy, Fruity Yogurt

## 82 Calories

## Ingredients

42g (1½ oz) fat-free natural Greek yogurt

4g (2 level tsp) ground almonds

Pinch of cinnamon

28g (1oz) blueberries

Stevia to sweeten if required

## Method

- Stir almonds & cinnamon into yogurt
- Mix in blueberries, adding stevia to taste
- Transfer to small bowl & eat with a teaspoon

# Baked Bean Breakfast

## 98 calories

### Ingredients

1 small slice wholemeal bread

56g (2 oz) canned baked beans

### Method

- Toast both sides of bread
- Place baked beans in microwavable container & cover
- Heat for 1 - 1½ minutes in microwave then stir
- Spoon onto toast & serve on an attractive small plate

# Fruity Refresher

## 87 Calories

## Ingredients

150 ml (5 fl. oz) water

42g (1½ oz) frozen pineapple chunks

½ small banana

42g (1½ oz) blueberries

14g (½ oz) watercress

Thin slice orange

## Method

- Pour water into a blender
- Add pineapple, banana & blueberries
- Put in watercress
- Blend until smooth
- Pour into tall glass
- Add orange slice
- Sip slowly

# Nutty Apple

## 105 Calories

### Ingredients

I medium apple

1 tsp crunchy peanut butter

### Method

- Cut apple into quarters, core & slice
- Top each quarter with a little peanut butter
- Mindfully munch each bite

# Smooth Carrot, Apple & Beetroot

## 124 Calories

## Ingredients

120 ml (4 fl.oz) carrot juice

1 small cooked peeled beetroot

1 small ripe unpeeled apple

Crushed Ice

## Method

- Core & slice apple finely
- Chop beetroot into pieces
- Pour carrot juice into a blender
- Add apple, beetroot & ice
- Blend until smooth
- Pour into glass, serve & savour each drop

# Banana with Chocolate

## 117 Calories

## Ingredients

1 tbsp semi-sweet chocolate chips

1 tbsp fat-free natural yogurt

Half a banana

## Method

- Put chocolate chips into small bowl
- Melt in microwave
- Mix yogurt into melted chocolate
- Cut banana into thin slices
- Top with mixture
- Savour slowly!

# Spicy Porridge

## 130 Calories

## Ingredients

20g (¾ oz) porridge oats

120 ml (4 fl.oz) almond milk

Pinch of cinnamon

Pinch of grated nutmeg

Pinch of salt

½ tsp mixed peel

1 tsp sultanas

## Method

- Pour oats into small saucepan
- Add almond milk
- Over gentle heat stir until creamy & you have your required consistency
- Sprinkle in cinnamon & nutmeg
- Add pinch of salt & stevia
- Stir in mixed peel & sultanas
- Scoop into a bowl to serve

# Cheesy Toast

## 111 Calories

## Ingredients

I small slice wholemeal bread

28g (1 oz) low fat cottage cheese

1 tsp cinnamon

## Method

- Preheat grill to medium
- Toast bread on both sides
- Spoon cottage cheese onto it
- Sprinkle with cinnamon
- Place on grill pan
- Cook, watching until the cottage cheese bubbles & begins to brown slightly
- Transfer to plate & eat whilst hot

# Giant Mushroom Munch

## 78 Calories

## Ingredients

2 large (Portobello) mushrooms

1 small garlic clove, peeled

1 tsp freshly chopped parsley

1 medium orange pepper

1 tsp olive oil

Ground black pepper

## Method

- Preheat grill to medium
- Brush mushrooms to clean & remove stalks
- Crush garlic clove, deseed pepper & chop
- Mix mushroom stalks in bowl with parsley, chopped pepper, garlic & oil
- Put mushrooms with skin uppermost onto grill pan & grill for 4 minutes
- Turn mushrooms over & divide garlic & pepper mixture onto open sides
- Season with a little pepper
- Grill for another 5 - 6 minutes before serving

# Creamy Strawberry Crackers

## 64 Calories

### Ingredients

2 low fat crackers

1 tbsp low fat cream cheese (e.g. Philadelphia light)

28g (1 oz) strawberries

### Method

- Place crackers on small plate
- Top with cream cheese
- Pop on strawberries (sliced if large)
- Enjoy!

# Smooth & Fruity

## 133 calories

## Ingredients

84 (3 oz) low fat cottage cheese

84g (3 oz) canned, drained pineapple chunks

2 tsp wheat germ

## Method

- Spoon cottage cheese into a smallish wide topped glass
- Add pineapple chunks
- Sprinkle decoratively with wheat germ
- Eat with a teaspoon

# Bacon with Egg & Tomato

## 143 Calories

## Ingredients

1-cal spray

1 lean rasher of bacon

1 small egg

1 medium tomato

Ground black pepper

## Method

- Preheat grill to medium
- Slice tomato in half & place on non-stick foil lined grill tray
- Add bacon & grill with tomato for approx. 4 minutes
- Spray non-stick lidded frying pan with 3 sprays of oil, cover before heating on very low heat
- Turn bacon over & continue cooking for approx. further 3 minutes
- Break egg into frying pan & cover with lid (this avoids the sneezed-on appearance!)
- Cook for approx. 3 minutes

- Remove egg from pan & slide onto plate with bacon & tomato halves
- Sprinkle lightly with black pepper before serving

# LUNCHES

# Cottage Cheese lunch

## 188 Calories

## Ingredients

2 small slices wholemeal bread

56g.(2 oz) natural cottage cheese

2 cherry tomatoes

4 sprigs parsley

Ground black pepper

## Method

- Place bread slices on a plate
- Spread with cottage cheese
- Cut each slice into half
- Halve tomatoes
- Top each half of bread with a tomato half & parsley sprig
- Sprinkle with pepper
- Enjoy mindfully!

# Roasted Vegetable Mix

## 71 Calories

### Ingredients

1 small plum tomato, chopped into small chunks

½ small sweet or red onion, sliced thinly

42g (1½ oz) mushrooms, sliced thickly

1 tsp olive oil

2 tsp red wine vinegar

1 tsp fresh basil, finely chopped

Ground black pepper

### Method

- Preheat oven to $200^0$C/$400^0$F/Gas mark 6
- In a large bowl, mix  tomato chunks with onion & mushroom slices
- Add oil, vinegar, basil & mix thoroughly with vegetables
- Season with black pepper to taste
- Line a baking tray with non-stick foil
- Spread vegetable mixture onto tray

- Roast vegetables until onion slices are browned & rest of vegetables are tender, keeping track when they are cooking to ensure that vegetables do not shrivel up (approx.15 - 20 minutes)
- Serve hot

# Barbecue-Flavoured Courgettes

## 123 Calories

### Ingredients

1 medium courgette

1 tbsp low calorie barbecue sauce

2 tbsp low fat grated cheddar cheese

1 tsp chopped coriander

1 small spring onion

2 sprigs parsley

### Method

- Chop off ends of courgette & discard
- Chop spring onion
- Use fork to prick courgette in several places
- Put on plate in microwave for 2 minutes
- Turn & microwave for 1 – 2 minutes
- Allow to cool for approx. 5 minutes
- Halve courgette by slicing lengthways
- Top each half evenly with cheese & sprinkle with sauce

- Microwave for 20 – 30 seconds until cheese melts before removing from microwave
- Top both halves with chopped onion
- Decorate with parsley
- Serve

# Roasted Red peppers & Cauliflower

## 84 Calories

## Ingredients

½ red pepper

1 clove garlic, peeled

100g (3½ oz) cauliflower florets

1 tsp olive oil

1- cal olive oil spray

2 tbsp shredded fresh basil leaves

Ground black pepper

## Method

- Preheat oven to $230^0C/450^0F$/Gas mark 8
- Slice red pepper
- Crush garlic
- Line shallow baking tray with non-stick alumium foil
- Spread pepper slices & cauliflower florets onto tray
- Drizzle olive oil over vegetables
- Coat with 4 squirts of spray

- Season with basil 7 black pepper
- Roast until vegetables are tender (approx. 12 minutes)

# Ricotta Cheese with Cherries & Almonds

## 150 Calories

### Ingredients

2 tbsp fat-free ricotta cheese

168 g (6 oz) frozen, stoneless cherries

1 tbsp toasted slice almonds

### Method

- Put cherries in small microwavable container & heat until warm (approx. 1½ minutes)
- Transfer to small bowl
- Place ricotta cheese over cherries
- Sprinkle with almonds & serve

# Tangy Snack

## 201 Calories

## Ingredients

1 slice crusty wholewheat bread

7g (¼ oz) mature cheddar cheese

10 cherry tomatoes

6 olives

## Method

- Cut bread into small pieces
- Slice cheese thinly
- De-stone & slice olives
- Put bread pieces, cheese, tomatoes & olive slices into a bowl
- Serve

# Spicy Omelette

## 130 Calories

### Ingredients

1 medium egg

2 cherry tomatoes

½ small green chilli

1 spring onion

14g (½ oz) low-fat grated cheese

Ground black pepper

½ tsp butter

2 tsp Mexican salsa

### Method

- Slice tomatoes, chilli &spring onion
- Heat non-stick frying pan on medium heat
- Break egg into bowl & add cheese
- Beat egg & cheese together with a fork
- Season with pepper
- Heat butter in frying pan
- Add chilli & onion & stir

- Pour in egg & cheese mix into frying pan, covering it evenly
- Add tomato slices to one half, cook until set
- Fold other half over the half with tomato
- Cook until both sides are nicely browned
- Remove omelette from pan & drizzle salsa over it
- Serve

# Sweet Tomato Treat

## 75 Calories

## Ingredients

1-cal olive oil spray

1 tsp olive oil

1 tbsp chopped spring onions

150g (5½ oz) cherry tomatoes

2 tbsp chopped parsley

Ground black pepper

## Method

- Use 5 sprays to coat frying pan & place on medium heat
- Mix tsp olive oil into chopped spring onion, add to frying pan & cook until soft, approx. 2 minutes
- Add in tomatoes & cook for about 5 more minutes, until softened
- Remove from heat, place on plate, add parsley & stir
- Season with pepper & serve

# Cottage Cheese with Onion & Peppers

## 100 Calories

## Ingredients

112g (4 oz) low-fat cottage cheese

168g (6 oz) yellow, green &orange peppers

3 small spring onions

Ground pepper

Tiny pinch of salt

## Method

- Chop peppers & spring onions finely
- Put cottage cheese into a bowl & add peppers
- Stir in chopped spring onions
- Season with salt & pepper
- Give it another brief stir
- It's ready to serve

# Cauliflower Soup

## 125 Calories

## Ingredients

240 ml (8 fl. oz) vegetable stock

1 tbsp lemon juice

½ medium cauliflower

1-cal olive oil spray

1 tbsp chopped spring onion

Pinch of nutmeg

Pinch of ground black pepper

## Method

- Put stock & lemon juice into large saucepan & heat on high setting until it begins to boil
- Meanwhile, cut cauliflower into florets
- Immediately lower heat to medium, add cauliflower florets to stock, partially cover & continue cooking until tender, approx 10 minutes

- Spray non-stick frying pan with 5 sprays to coat & cook chopped spring onion until tender, approx. 4 minutes
- Stir spring onion into soup mix
- Pour into a blender & purée until smooth
- Transfer to bowl & serve

# Colourful Coleslaw

## 61 Calories

### Ingredients

112g (4 oz) red cabbage

¼ small white onion

1 small carrot

2 tbsp very light mayonnaise (eg. Hellmann's)

Small pinch of ground black pepper

### Method

- Shred red cabbage
- Chop onion & carrots
- Put cabbage & onion into a bowl
- Mix in mayonnaise & sprinkle on pepper
- Stir well before serving

# Creamy Bagel

## 97 Calories

## Ingredients

Mini bagel

2 tsp low fat cream cheese

2 sprigs parsley

## Method

- Cut bagel into half & toast
- Spread with cream cheese
- Top each half with parsley

# SUPPERS

# Tortilla Treat

## 153 Calories

## Ingredients

2 corn tortillas

2 tablespoons grated low fat cheddar cheese

1 tablespoon salsa

120 ml (4fl.oz) liquid egg substitute

1-cal olive oil spray

## Method

- Put cheese & salsa onto tortillas; set to one side
- Coat small non-stick frying pan with 4 sprays.
- Heat gently on medium heat
- Pour in egg substitute & stir constantly until cooked (approx.90 seconds)
- Heat topped tortillas in a microwave until cheese melts (approx.30 seconds)
- Scoop scrambled egg evenly onto each tortilla
- Savour them slowly

# Bulgur wheat salad

## 326 Calories

## Ingredients

63g (2¼ oz) bulgur wheat

150ml (5 fl.oz) water

Small pinch of salt

Ground black pepper

84g (3oz) cherry tomatoes

3 spring onions

5 sprigs parsley

¼ cucumber

1 orange pepper

2 tsp olive oil

1tbsp balsamic vinegar

5 round lettuce leaves

1tbsp. feta cheese, crumbled

## Method

- Boil water, salted to taste, in small saucepan
- Remove from heat
- Pour in bulgur wheat & give it a quick stir
- Cover with lid
- Leave for 20 minutes before draining off any excess liquid
- Transfer to bowl & fluff lightly with a fork, before putting aside to cool
- Halve cherry tomatoes
- Chop spring onions & parsley
- Slice cucumber & pepper
- Place cooled bulgur wheat, with chopped & sliced vegetables & feta cheese, in large bowl
- Add vinegar, olive oil & pepper & combine thoroughly
- Arrange lettuce leaves to overlap on plate
- Serve bulgur & vegetable on bed of lettuce

# Baked Cod with Vegetables

## 248 Calories

## Ingredients

150g (5½ oz) cod fillet, skinless

½  orange pepper

½ yellow pepper

½ red onion

½ courgette

56g (2 oz) cherry tomatoes

2 black olives

Juice & zest of ¼ lemon

2 tsp fresh thyme leaves

1-cal spray

Ground black pepper

Pinch of salt

## Method

- Preheat oven to 200°C/400°F/Gas mark 6.
- Line baking tray with non-stick alumium foil
- Chop peppers, onion & courgette
- Spread them onto baking tray
- Coat with 4 sprays of oil
- Season with salt & pepper
- Roast for approx 10 minutes
- Put cod fillet on top of vegetables
- Season with a little salt and pepper & spray 3 times with oil
- Surround fish with tomatoes, olives and sprinkle with lemon zest
- Squeeze lemon juice over them.
- Sprinkle with herbs
- Bake for approx.8 minutes, until the cod is thoroughly cooked.
- Slice & de-stone olives to decorate food
- Serve while piping hot

# Steak with Mushrooms & Tomatoes

## 247 Calories

## Ingredients

100g (3½ oz) lean sirloin steak

Ground black pepper

Pinch of salt

84g (3 oz) mushrooms

1-cal olive oil spray

227g (8 oz) canned chopped tomatoes

## Method

- Remove steak from fridge approx. half an hour before using to allow it to reach room temperature to avoid it ending up tough after cooking
- Preheat grill to medium high heat
- Pat steak dry on each side with paper towelling
- Sprinkle both sides with salt & pepper
- Place steak on grill pan
- Cook for approx.4 minutes on each side (length of time will obviously depend on how you like your steak)

- Spray mushrooms twice with oil & add to grill pan halfway through cooking
- Put tomatoes into microwaveable container, cover & heat in microwave for 1½ minutes
- Place steak on plate & top with mushrooms & tomatoes
- Serve

# Beef & Broccoli with Rice

## 335 Calories

**Ingredients**

60g (2 oz) long-grained rice

60g (2 oz) lean beef

1-cal olive oil spray

2 cloves garlic, peeled

2 spring onions

½ tsp ground coriander

½ tsp cumin

Pinch of ground black pepper

100g (3½ oz) broccoli florets

70g (2½ oz) tomatoes

**Method**

- Cook rice in pan of boiling water for 10 – 15 minutes
- Meanwhile, slice beef into strips, crush garlic, chop onions & halve tomatoes

- Drain cooked rice & rinse with boiling water to remove excess starch.
- Return rice to pan, cover with lid & place to one side
- Coat non-stick frying pan with 5 sprays oil & heat on high heat
- Sauté garlic with spring onions for 1 minute
- Add coriander, cumin, pepper & beef
- Cook for approx.3 minutes until beef is cooked through
- Add broccoli & tomatoes
- Lower heat to medium & cook for 3 further minutes
- Serve the mixture over rice

# Moroccan Couscous Supper

## 238 Calories

## Ingredients

227g (8 oz) can chopped tomatoes

½ tsp crushed coriander seeds

½ tsp crushed cumin seeds

300 ml (10 fl. oz) water

1 medium peeled carrot

1 medium leek

1 courgette

100g ((3½ oz) drained chickpeas

½ tsp turmeric

Ground black pepper

Salt

28g (1 oz) wholewheat couscous

75 ml (2½ fl.oz) boiling water

A few coriander leaves

## Method

- Preheat oven to 180°C/350°F/Gas mark 4
- Chop carrot
- Slice leek & courgettes
- Heat a heavy-based saucepan over a medium heat
- Put in coriander & cumin seeds & stir for approx. 20 seconds until they release their aroma
- Pour in chopped tomatoes & 300 ml water & bring to boiling point
- Add carrot, leek & courgette & chickpeas
- Stir in turmeric & season with pepper & salt
- Transfer mixture to casserole & cover
- Put into oven for approx. 1 hour or until vegetables are tender
- Put couscous into bowl, pour over 75 ml boiling water, stir well & cover
- Leave for 5 minutes until soft, giving the occasional stir
- Place oven-cooked mixture on plate & garnish with coriander leaves
- Serve hot with couscous

# Saucy Meatfree Burgers

## 229 Calories

## Ingredients

112g (4 oz) canned crushed tomatoes

¼ tsp dried mixed herbs

2 frozen soya meatfree burger

4 thick slices aubergine

1-cal olive oil spray

2 sprigs parsley

## Method

- Preheat grill to medium & place burgers on grill pan
- Cook for 10 – 12 minutes, turning occasionally
- Whilst they are cooking, coat a frying pan on medium heat with 4 sprays of oil
- Put in aubergine slices & cook until golden brown, 2 – 3 minutes per side
- Pour tomatoes into microwavable bowl & mix in herbs to make sauce

- Cover & microwave sauce until piping hot, approx. 20 seconds
- Place a burger on serving plate, top with aubergine slice, add spoonful of sauce, top with another aubergine slice then spoon on another dollop of sauce.
- Repeat above instruction with the other burger.
- Cover layered burgers with the rest of sauce
- Garnish with parsley
- Eat with a calorie-free smile!

# Grilled Haddock with Courgettes

## 212 Calories

## Ingredients

126g (4½ oz) haddock fillet

56g (2 oz) baby courgettes

1 tsp olive oil

56g (2 oz) tomato & chilli pasta sauce

Pinch of ground black pepper

Tiny pinch of salt

6 basil leaves

## Method

- Heat grill to medium
- Slice courgettes into halves
- Line grill pan with non-stick cooking foil
- Place haddock & courgettes onto pan & drizzle olive oil over them
- Grill for approx. 15 minutes, until fish & courgettes are cooked, turning courgettes half way through

- Tear basil leaves
- Cover sauce & microwave for 1 minute
- Transfer haddock & courgettes to plate & add sauce
- Sprinkle with basil & serve

# Stir-fried Chicken with Cashew Nuts

## 300 Calories

**Ingredients**

14g (½ oz) cashew nuts

1-cal olive oil

1 yellow pepper

1 red onion

112g (4oz) chicken breast, skinless

56g (2 oz) tenderstem broccoli

1 tsp grated ginger

1 garlic clove, peeled

1 tbsp water

1 tbsp sweet chilli sauce

1 tbsp soy sauce

100g ((3½ oz) Zero Noodles (freely available in USA & now reaching UK via health stores)

# Method

- Deseed & chop pepper
- Slice onion & crush garlic
- Cut chicken & broccoli into small pieces
- Place a wok on medium-high heat for a few seconds, until hot.
- Add cashew nuts & stir for 30 seconds until golden, before removing from heat & setting to one side
- Coat the wok with 5 sprays of oil, add pepper & onion
- Fry for 1 minute before adding chicken & stir-frying for 3 minutes until brown & nearly cooked
- Add broccoli, ginger & garlic, stir for 1 minute
- Add water, cover pan & cook for 2 minutes
- Rinse noodles with warm water, place in pan of boiling water & cook for 3-5 minutes
- Pour chilli & soy sauces into stir- fry, heat for a further minute
- Sprinkle on cashew nuts & turn off heat
- Drain noodles before adding to stir- fry.

# Tasty Tuna Salad

## 319 Calories

**Ingredients**

1small red onion

2 tbsp balsamic vinegar

200g (7 oz) total combined weight of raw or cooked vegetables below:-

> Chopped green beans
>
> Sliced radishes
>
> Cauliflower & broccoli florets
>
> Sliced carrot
>
> Sliced cucumber
>
> Chopped asparagus

90g (3 ¼ oz) canned tuna, in oil

Ground black pepper to taste

6 large round lettuce leaves

## Method

- Slice onion thinly & marinate in vinegar for minimum of 30 minutes
- Arrange lettuce leaves overlapping slightly on serving plate
- In large bowl mix onion with all the rest of above ingredients
- Spoon onto bed of lettuce

# Turkey with Wedges

## 218 Calories

## Ingredients

112g (4 oz) Potatoes

112g (4 oz) raw minced turkey

1 small garlic clove, peeled

1 spring onion

1 tsp chopped lemon thyme

Pinch of ground black pepper

Small pinch of salt

4 large lettuce leaves

Parsley sprig to garnish

1-cal olive oil

## Method

- Preheat oven to 220°C/425°F/Gas mark 7
- Cut potatoes into wedges

- Trim & chop spring onion
- Crush garlic
- In a bowl, mix onion, garlic, lemon thyme salt & pepper with minced turkey
- Shape mixture into a burger & chill for around 30 minutes
- Use 4 sprays of oil on an oven tray
- Put wedges onto tray & cook for approx 35 minutes, turning occasionally
- 15 minutes before wedges are cooked, spray burger once on each side & brush over gently
- Heat small frying pan over medium heat & fry burger for approx. 4 minutes per side until nicely browned
- Arrange lettuce leaves on plate
- Place turkey burger in the centre & cooked potato wedges around edge of lettuce bed
- Top with parsley & serve

# Spicy Chicken

## 180 Calories

## Ingredients

1 tbsp chipotle chilli paste or adjust to your taste

84g (3 oz) chicken breast

154g (5½ oz) vegetable stir-fry mix

1-cal olive oil spray

## Method

- Cut chicken into strips
- Put chipotle chilli paste with chicken strips into a bowl & stir thoroughly until well mixed
- Set aside for an hour to marinate
- Spray a wok with 3 sprays of oil, heat on medium setting & fry chicken, whilst stirring until cooked, 3 – 5 minutes
- Remove chicken & set aside
- Spray wok again twice then stir-fry vegetable mix for approx. 2 minutes on medium heat
- Return chicken to wok stirring into vegetable mix & cook for 3 minutes
- Serve